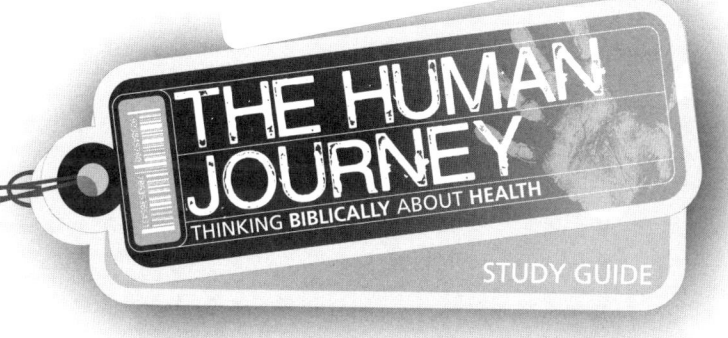

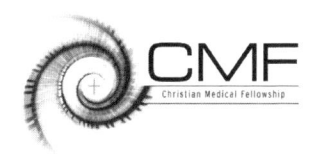

THE HUMAN JOURNEY
THINKING BIBLICALLY ABOUT HEALTH

STUDY GUIDE

CMF
Christian Medical Fellowship

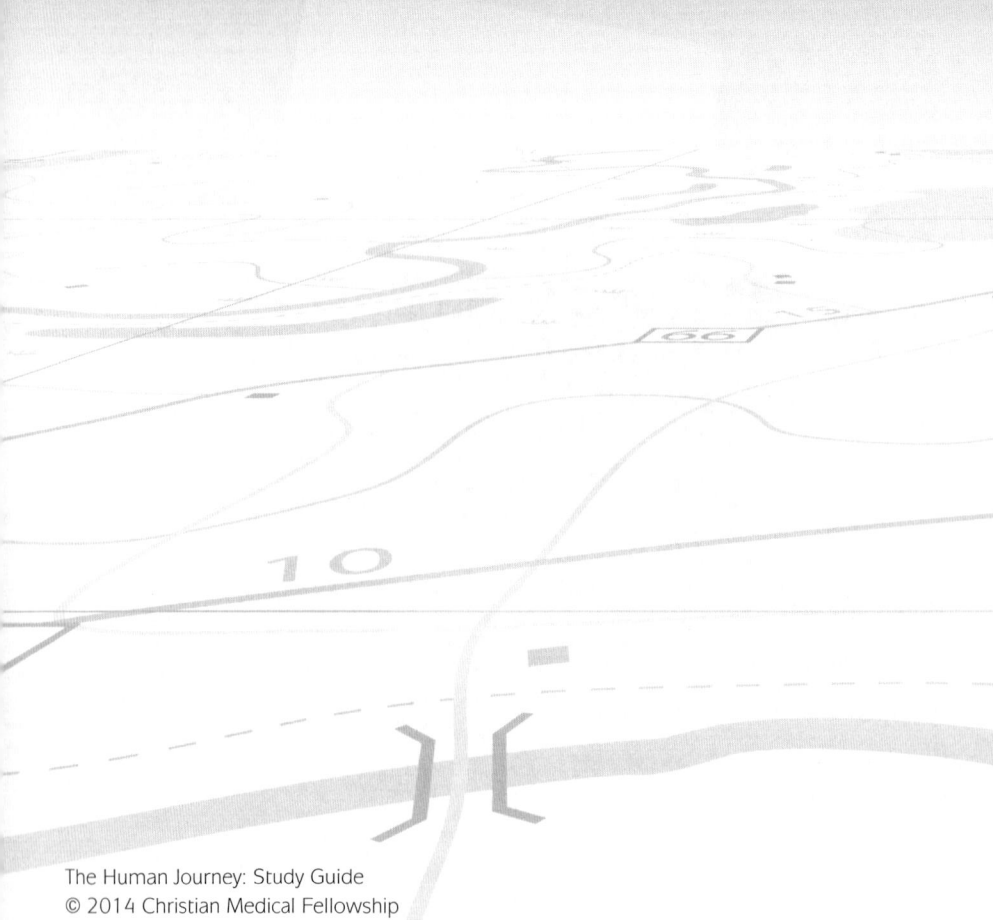

The Human Journey: Study Guide
© 2014 Christian Medical Fellowship
Christian Medical Fellowship has asserted its rights under the Copyright,
Design and Patents Act, 1988, to be identified as Author of this work.

Published by Christian Medical Fellowship
6 Marshalsea Road, London SE1 1HL, UK
www.cmf.org.uk

All rights reserved. No part of this publication may be reproduced or transmitted in any form or by any means, electronic or mechanical, including photocopy, recording or any information storage and retrieval system, without permission in writing from the publisher.

ISBN 978-0-906747-59-9

Design: S2 Design & Advertising
Printed by Stanley L Hunt Printers Ltd

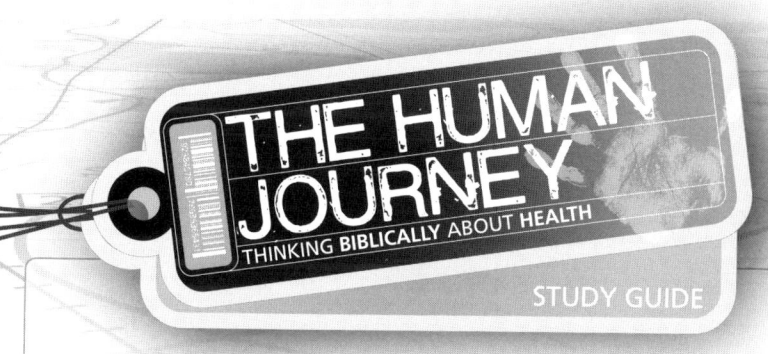

THE HUMAN JOURNEY
THINKING BIBLICALLY ABOUT HEALTH
STUDY GUIDE

Contents

Introduction	05
Humanity: What does it mean to be human?	06
Start of Life: When does life begin?	12
Marriage & Sexuality: What is marriage for?	18
Physical Health: How should I live?	26
Mental Health: Am I supposed to feel like this?	32
End of Life: How should life end?	38
New Technologies: Are we playing God?	44
Global Health: Who is my neighbour?	50

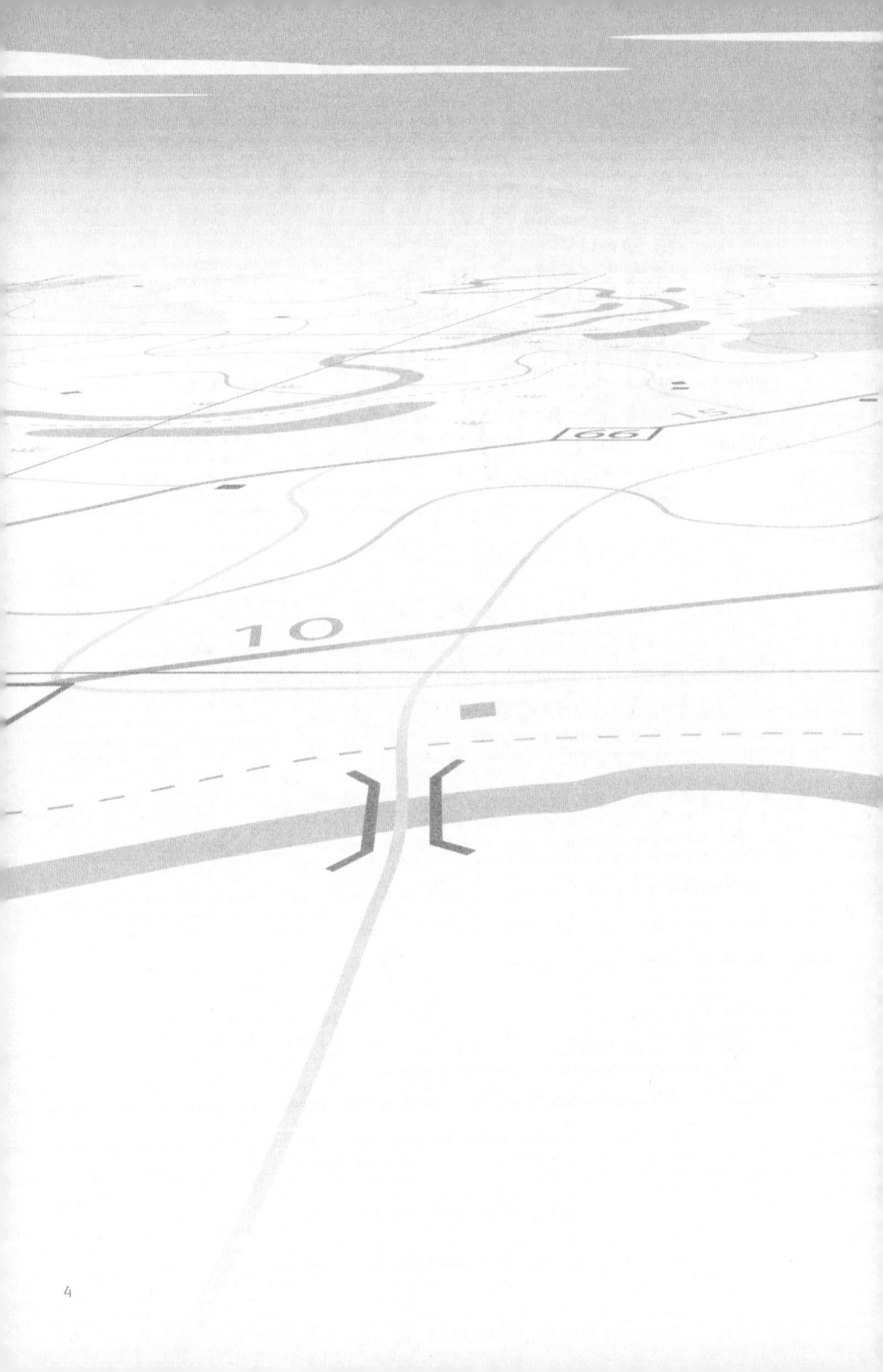

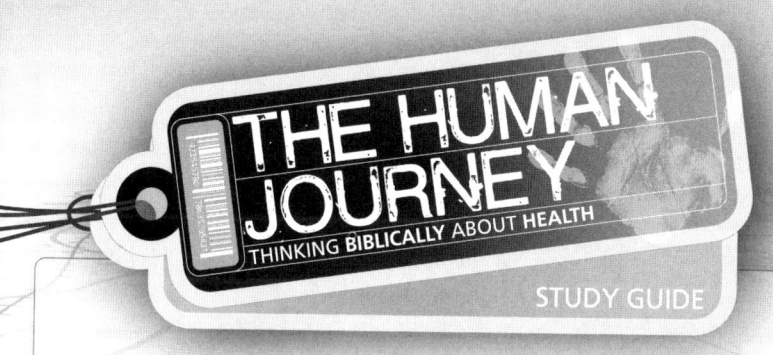

THE HUMAN JOURNEY
THINKING BIBLICALLY ABOUT HEALTH
STUDY GUIDE

Introduction

Welcome to The Human Journey! This material flows out of the firm belief that God's word contains timeless wisdom to help us think about our own health and the health of those around us.

We have chosen the eight key topics because we think that, in one way or another, they encompass almost all the most important health-related issues. We believe the Bible can address these areas because the same God who made us has revealed his will for our lives in his word. Scripture does not answer every question directly, but it leads us towards principles that help us to address the issues of our age.

The course is accompanied by several additional resources to help you explore issues further and engage with others:

- *The Human Journey* **book**, expanding on the teaching contained in the videos.

- **Website**, containing further resources for each topic: *www.humanjourney.org.uk*

- **Social media pages** for you to engage with us and others exploring these issues:
    - Facebook: *facebook.com/thehumanjourney*
    - Twitter: *@thehumanjourney* or *twitter.com/thehumanjourney*

We hope that this course will leave you excited about the whole Bible, more amazed about Christ's great work and all that it means and more confident about how to apply God's word to your life.

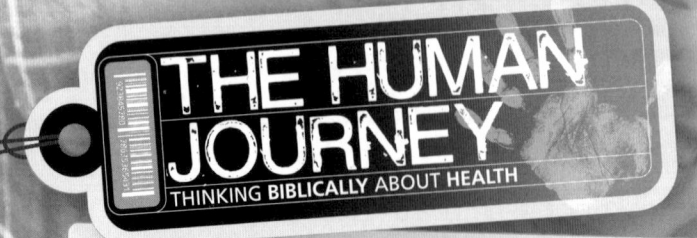

THE HUMAN JOURNEY
THINKING BIBLICALLY ABOUT HEALTH

HUMANITY:
WHAT DOES IT MEAN TO BE HUMAN?

SESSION AIM
To explore what being made 'in the image of God' means, how humans are different from animals, and to examine the effects of sin on all humanity.

ICEBREAKER
Can you think of a time when you've been reminded about how precious human life is? What made it so special?

○ WATCH THE DVD

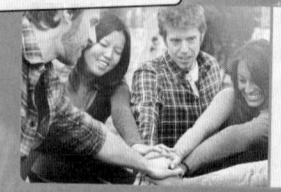

▷ HUMANITY:
WHAT DOES IT MEAN
TO BE HUMAN?

Opening verses: Psalm 8:4–8

DVD KEY POINTS

After centuries of debate, the question of what it means to be human is still hotly disputed today.

Animal rights and 'Speciesism'

Made in God's image

The bearer of the image of God belongs to God (Matthew 22:15–22)

This special status has six dimensions:
- Representative (Genesis 1:28)
- Spiritual (Genesis 2:7)
- Moral (Genesis 2:16–17)
- Immortal (Genesis 2:17)
- Relational (Genesis 2:18)
- Creative (Genesis 2:19)

Secular models of humanity

Spirit, soul and body

The Fall (Genesis 3)

Relationships are broken:
- With God
- With one another
- With creation

Summary

Humans are unique because we are made in the image of God. This conveys special responsibilities and marks humans off from animals. But due to the Fall, humans are fatally flawed and relationships at all levels are distorted. All that was lost in the Fall, however, will be restored through Christ.

THE HUMAN JOURNEY

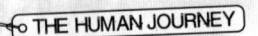

EXPLORE

Key passages: Genesis 1:26–31; Psalm 8.
Use these, and any other relevant passages you can think of, to help you discuss the following questions together.

1 How does society generally view human nature? Why do you think this is?

2 The video highlighted six aspects of what it means to be made 'in the image of God'. Can you think of any other ways that humans reflect God?

3 *'Humans are no different to animals.'* What do you think of this statement? What does Scripture teach about this?

HUMANITY

4 How has the Fall (Genesis 3) affected humans? In what ways have you seen these effects in yourself and others? (See eg. Romans 1:28–32, 3:9–18)

5 If humans are made in the image of God, how might this shape our attitudes to those who are weak and vulnerable, or who are looked down on in our society?

6 All humans are fallen and affected by sin. How does Jesus offer us hope? (eg Romans 8:29; 1 Corinthians 15:49; 2 Corinthians 3:18)

THE HUMAN JOURNEY

GO FURTHER

- Is there someone you know in your church or circle of friends who is vulnerable or in need? How could you encourage them, help them and remind them that they too are made in God's image?

- Before the next session, read Psalm 139 and use this to reflect on the value and preciousness of life in God's sight (this will also help you prepare for the next session).

PRAY

Pray together or in smaller groups about what you've learned in this session. You may like to use these points as a guide:

- Thank God for the unique blessing of being made in his image.

- Pray for wisdom to carry out the responsibilities we have as his people.

- Pray that we would see the image of God in all people, and value them as we should.

- Thank God for sending his Son, Jesus Christ who was fully human and fully God, to rescue and restore the relationship broken by the Fall.

- Ask God to help us be committed to standing up for and serving those who are most vulnerable in society.

GLOSSARY

- **Reductionism**: A philosophical position which holds that a complex system is nothing but the sum of its parts.

- **Speciesism**: A term used to argue that privileging one species over another (eg assigning greater value to humans than animals) is a prejudice similar to racism or sexism.

- **Taxonomy**: A field of science that involves the description, identification, naming and classification of living organisms.

To continue thinking about the topics raised in this session read chapter one of *The Human Journey* book: 'Humanity: What does it mean to be human?'

More resources on Humanity are available at *www.humanjourney.org.uk*

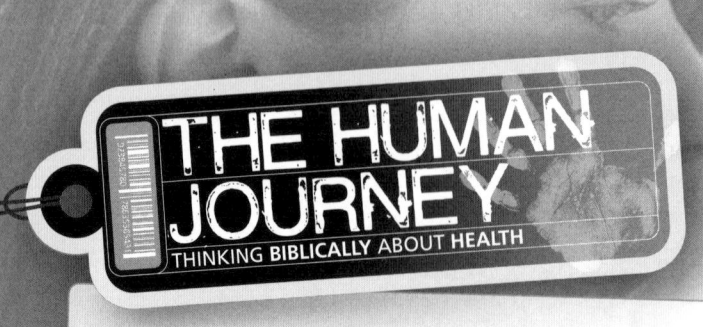

THE HUMAN JOURNEY
THINKING BIBLICALLY ABOUT HEALTH

START OF LIFE
WHEN DOES LIFE BEGIN?

SESSION AIM
To explore secular and biblical perspectives on when human life begins and examine our responsibility as Christians to value life from its very beginning.

ICEBREAKER
Discuss what you have observed about human life and its value from close friends or family (or personally) going through a pregnancy.

WATCH THE DVD

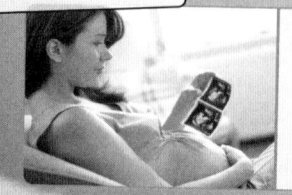

▷ START OF LIFE:
   WHEN DOES LIFE BEGIN?
   Opening verses: Psalm 139:13–16

START OF LIFE

DVD KEY POINTS

From what point does the value of human life exist?

The answer we come to will affect how we deal with many important medical decisions:
- Abortion
- Medical Research
- Contraception
- Embryonic cloning and some three-parent embryo techniques
- Fertility treatments

Starting points
Different people choose to draw the line of humanity at different points:
- Fertilisation
- Implantation
- Organ development
- Nervous system
- Quickening
- Viability
- First breath

Clues from the Bible
There are many references in Scripture to human life before the time of birth.

'For you created my inmost being; you knit me together in my mother's womb' (Psalm 139:13–14).

Psalm 139 expresses three important truths:
- Creation
- Communion
- Continuity

Summary
The biblical testimony about life before birth leads us to the conclusion that from the time of conception a valuable human life exists. The developing human being in the womb is also our neighbour: made in the image of God and worthy of the utmost respect, wonder, empathy, and protection.

THE HUMAN JOURNEY

EXPLORE

Key passages: Psalm 139:13–16; Luke 1:39–45.
Use these, and any other relevant passages you can think of, to help you discuss the following questions.

1. The video outlined the main positions on when life begins. Did any of them surprise you? Why?

2. What principles can we draw from the Bible about how we should view human life before birth?

3 What practical implications might these passages have for your view of:

A. Abortion

B. Screening embryos for Down's syndrome and other genetic conditions

C. Research that uses embryos

THE HUMAN JOURNEY

GO FURTHER

- Think of something you could do to raise awareness of the value and sanctity of human life before birth. You could write a letter to your MP or elected representative or post something on social media, or just talk to people you know.

PRAY

Pray together about what you've learned in this session. You may like to use these points as a guide:

- Pray for a greater sense of awe and reverence towards the God who created us all.

- Thank God for the gift of human life and pray that he will help us protect and preserve it to the best of our abilities.

- Pray for courage and strength to stand up and speak out when challenged about the status of human life before birth.

START OF LIFE

GLOSSARY

- **Embryo**: The developing baby from the moment an egg and sperm fuse until eight weeks gestation in the womb.

- **Fertilisation**: The event that occurs when a sperm meets and fuses with a mature egg (also called conception).

- **Fetus**: The developing baby in the womb from eight weeks to birth.

- **Implantation**: After fertilisation, the egg travels down the Fallopian tube and attaches to the inner lining of the uterus.

- **Quickening**: When the baby can be felt kicking and moving by the mother.

To continue thinking about the topics raised in this session read chapter two of *The Human Journey* book: Start of Life – When does life begin?

More resources on Start of Life are available at *www.humanjourney.org.uk*

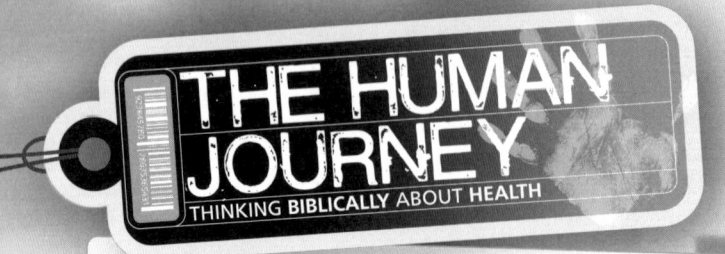

THE HUMAN JOURNEY
THINKING BIBLICALLY ABOUT HEALTH

MARRIAGE & SEXUALITY
WHAT IS MARRIAGE FOR?

SESSION AIM
To understand God's design for marriage, the blessings marriage brings and the risks of departing from this pattern.

ICEBREAKER
Share together about couples you know of who have been married for a long time. What do you think keeps them together?

▶ WATCH THE DVD

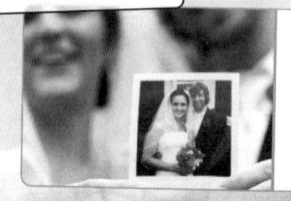

▷ MARRIAGE & SEXUALITY: WHAT IS MARRIAGE FOR?

Opening verses: Ephesians 5:25–30

MARRIAGE & SEXUALITY

DVD KEY POINTS

Healthy marriages are key to a healthy church and society.

The purpose of marriage
The Bible teaches that marriage provides:
- Companionship
- A context for sexual intimacy
- A stable environment for reproduction
- A nourishing environment for child rearing
- Security for marriage partners and family members

The most profound purpose is that marriage points to Christ's relationship with his people, the church.

The pattern of marriage
Genesis 2:24 teaches that marriage is to be:
- Unconditional
- Lifelong
- Exclusively monogamous
- Sexually intimate
- Heterosexual

The practice of marriage
Husbands and wives get different but complementary exhortations (Ephesians 5:23, 25).

The husband has a challenging role, because with headship comes accountability, responsibility and servanthood.

What about sex outside of marriage?
The New Testament places sex outside of marriage in the category of 'sexual immorality' (*porneia*).

Sexual sin is called a sin against the body (1 Corinthians 6:18). Our bodies belong to the Lord (1 Corinthians 6:19-20).

Summary
Christians – married or single – should celebrate, demonstrate, promote and protect the institution of marriage.

THE HUMAN JOURNEY

EXPLORE

Key passages: Genesis 2:23–24; Matthew 19:3–6; Ephesians 5:31–33

Use these, and any other relevant passages you can think of, to help you discuss the following questions.

1 What attitudes have you noticed towards marriage in society (outside the church)? How does this compare to the Bible's teaching on marriage?

2 Look again at Ephesians 5:21–33. In what ways is a husband to be like Christ? In what ways is a wife to be like the church? What are the differences? What dangers are there if either spouse distorts their role?

MARRIAGE & SEXUALITY

3 The Bible's teaching about 'submission' can be controversial. How does Ephesians 5:21 and the role of the husband described in Ephesians 5:25–30 help us to understand this idea better?

○ THE HUMAN JOURNEY

4 How might you answer someone who thinks that reserving sex for within marriage or that having to commit to one person for life is restrictive?

5 'Sex outside of marriage is disastrous and has disastrous consequences.' Do you think this is right? What consequences can follow from sex outside marriage?

MARRIAGE & SEXUALITY

6 As well as talking about marriage, Scripture addresses those who are single (eg 1 Corinthians 7:32–40). What are the challenges and benefits of being single?

7 How should churches support those who are not married?

THE HUMAN JOURNEY

GO FURTHER

- If you are married, think of ways you and your spouse could:

  - Improve your own marriage
  - Pray for and support couples who are engaged or considering marriage.

- If you are single, chat to a married couple you know and ask how you could pray for them and how they could pray for you.

PRAY

Pray together or in smaller groups about what you've learned in this session. You may like to use these points as a guide:

- Pray for your own marriage, or the marriages of friends you have, that Jesus Christ would be central.

- Pray for wisdom and peace for anyone you know who is struggling in their marriage.

- Pray for the awareness to know that our ultimate identity and value lies in Christ, not in whether we are single or married.

MARRIAGE & SEXUALITY

GLOSSARY

- **Cohabitation**: The practice of two unmarried people (a man and woman) who live together and have a sexual relationship or live as though married.

- **Monogamy**: The practice of having one husband or wife.

To continue thinking about the topics raised in this session read chapter three of *The Human Journey* book: Marriage & Sexuality – What is marriage for?

More resources on Marriage & Sexuality are available at *www.humanjourney.org.uk*

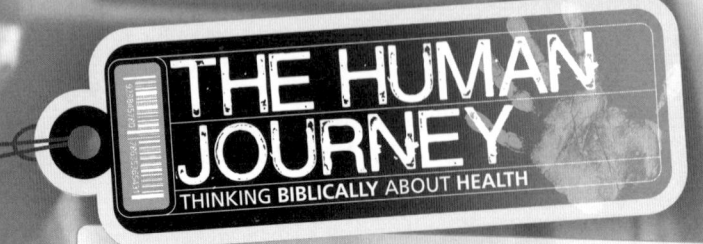

THE HUMAN JOURNEY
THINKING BIBLICALLY ABOUT HEALTH

PHYSICAL HEALTH
HOW SHOULD I LIVE?

SESSION AIM
To understand factors which affect physical health, and explore biblical principles about how we should view our bodies.

ICEBREAKER
Have you ever made an effort to get fit? What did you have to change about your lifestyle? Was it easy?

WATCH THE DVD

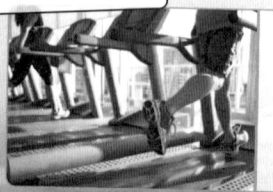

▷ PHYSICAL HEALTH: HOW SHOULD I LIVE?
   Opening verses: Philippians 3:17–21

PHYSICAL HEALTH

DVD KEY POINTS

Most people don't live longer than 70–90 years. Environment and availability of medical care can affect how long we live. We can't always control these, but we do have a lot of control over our lifestyle choices.

The five big killers
- Cancer
- Coronary heart disease
- Stroke
- Lung disease
- Liver disease

Improving our health
- Eat a healthy diet
- Maintain a healthy weight
- Stay physically active

A biblical perspective
- We are mortal (2 Corinthians 4:16–5:4)
- Illness is part of living in a fallen world (Genesis 3)
- We should treat our bodies with respect (1 Corinthians 6:19–20)

Alcohol in the Bible
There are warnings about alcohol the Old Testament (Noah and Lot, Genesis 9:20–23, 19:30–38) and the New Testament (Ephesians 5:18).

The Bible doesn't prohibit drinking alcohol, but does prohibit getting drunk.

Obesity
Obesity was not a major problem in the past, but Proverbs gives warnings about overeating (Proverbs 25:16, 28:7).

Summary
Our bodies are temples of the Holy Spirit. We must keep health in an eternal perspective. This life is only a shadow of what is to come, and the life that follows is infinitely more important.

THE HUMAN JOURNEY

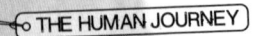

EXPLORE

> **Key passages:** 1 Thessalonians 5:4–8;
> 1 Corinthians 6:19–20; 8:1–13; Philippians 3:17–21
> Use these, and any other relevant passages you can think of, to help you discuss the following questions.

1 What views of the body and physical fitness are common in society? What is good and bad about these?

2 How much should Christians care about a body which is 'wasting away' (2 Corinthians 4:16). Why?

3 *'We shouldn't be surprised when we or our loved ones eventually develop some serious illness.'* What comfort does Scripture offer us in the face of this possibility? How could you encourage a loved one who became seriously ill?

4 What guidelines can we take from Scripture about:

A.   Recreational drugs

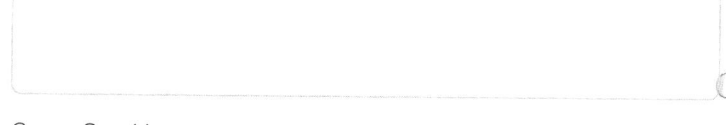

B.   Drinking alcohol

C.   Smoking

D.   Overeating

THE HUMAN JOURNEY

GO FURTHER

- What changes could you make to your lifestyle and diet to help improve your physical health?

- Think of ways you can encourage others to take their physical health more seriously. Perhaps you could be starting an exercise class at church, or run a healthy eating event.

PRAY

Pray together or in smaller groups about what you've learned in this session. You may like to use these points as a guide:

- Thank God that he has given each one of us a unique set of gifts and physical abilities.

- Pray for the strength and courage to be good stewards of our bodies so that we can use our gifts and abilities well.

- Pray for those who are stuck in physical addictions, that they would know the hope and healing of God in their lives.

PHYSICAL HEALTH

GLOSSARY

- **Body Mass Index**: A measure to determine if someone is a healthy weight for their height.

- **Obesity**: The condition of being very overweight, usually defined as having a Body Mass Index (BMI) in excess of 30.

To continue thinking about the topics raised in this session read chapter four of *The Human Journey* book: Physical Health – How should I live?

More resources on Physical Health are available at *www.humanjourney.org.uk*

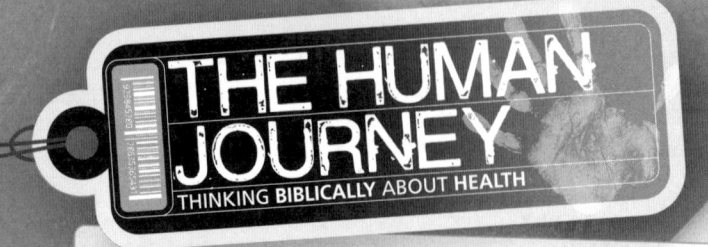

THE HUMAN JOURNEY
THINKING BIBLICALLY ABOUT HEALTH

MENTAL HEALTH
AM I SUPPOSED TO FEEL LIKE THIS?

SESSION AIM
To look at biblical principles about ways to keep ourselves mentally healthy, and explore how we can support those who are mentally ill.

ICEBREAKER
What do you usually do to lift your spirits on a bad day? Chat to a friend? Read the Bible? Eat chocolate?

○ WATCH THE DVD

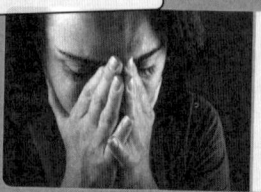

▷ MENTAL HEALTH:
AM I SUPPOSED TO FEEL LIKE THIS?
Opening verses: Philippians 4:8–9

MENTAL HEALTH

DVD KEY POINTS

Just as we will suffer from physical illnesses, many will also suffer from a mental illness at some time in their lives.

Being anxious or feeling low are not the same as having a psychiatric disorder or mental illness.

The church can help but real mental illness also needs the expertise of healthcare professionals.

The effects of the Fall
The Fall profoundly influences our mental health through our:
- Genes
- Environment
- Relationships
- Personal choices

What does the Bible say?
The clearest example of mental illness is Nebuchadnezzar (Daniel 4).

Jesus' death and resurrection changes us; nothing can separate us from God's love, we have a hope of future beyond the grave, and are in a loving community (the church).

Elijah's mental meltdown (1 Kings 19:1–21)
God's provides Elijah with:
- Rest, food and drink
- Reassurance of his love
- A fresh filling of his Spirit
- Reinforcements
- A new job to do

Summary
The Bible encourages us to think in constructive ways:
- Actively rejoicing in God's nature, truth and victory
- Being in continual conversation with him
- Choosing to give thanks in everything for all his blessings and promises.

But we should not turn our backs on proven, God-given, specialist care.

THE HUMAN JOURNEY

EXPLORE

Key passages: Psalm 42 and 43; Philippians 4:6–9
Use these, and any other relevant passages you can think of, to help you discuss the following questions.

1 What common attitudes are there to mental health issues in society? Why do you think this is?

2 How does the psalmist's language reveal his mental and emotional condition? (Psalm 42 and 43)

3 If this was a family member or friend, how could you support them?

MENTAL HEALTH

4 How does the psalmist speak to himself (Psalm 42:5, 11; 43:5)? How could this help?

5 The apostle Paul instructs us to 'rejoice in the Lord always' (Philippians 4:4). What do you think this means? What would this look like in practice?

6 How can Philippians 4:6–9 be helpful to someone struggling with depression? How must we be careful with passages like these?

THE HUMAN JOURNEY

GO FURTHER

- Think of ways you can support and pray for people in your church and community who struggle with their mental health. How can you and your church care for them better?

- Reflect on your own mental health. What steps can you take to maintain or improve a helpful and positive thought life? This might involve reading the Bible or talking with trusted friends or your church leaders.

PRAY

Pray together or in smaller groups about what you've learned in this session. You may like to use these points as a guide:

- Thank God for the eternal hope we have in him and the peace we can know which transcends all understanding.

- Pray for those you know of who are suffering a mental illness – pray for peace, healing and resilience.

- Pray for doctors, nurses and healthcare professionals who care for people suffering from mental illnesses that they would make wise, compassionate and life-affirming clinical decisions.

GLOSSARY

- **Cognitive Behavioural Therapy (CBT)**: A talking therapy used to help people change thoughts, feelings and behaviours that are causing them problems. It doesn't remove people's problems, but better equips them to cope.

- **Depression**: A mental illness or mood disorder which makes people feel sad and pessimistic. Symptoms include low mood, feelings of hopelessness, low self-esteem, lethargy and sleep problems.

- **Psychiatry**: The medical specialty that deals specifically with the disorders of the mind.

To continue thinking about the topics raised in this session read chapter five of *The Human Journey* book: Mental Health – Am I supposed to feel like this?

More resources on Mental Health are available at *www.humanjourney.org.uk*

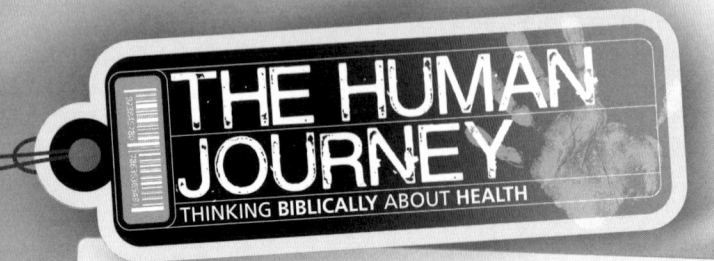

THE HUMAN JOURNEY
THINKING BIBLICALLY ABOUT HEALTH

END OF LIFE
HOW SHOULD LIFE END?

SESSION AIM
To explore changing attitudes to the end of life, and apply biblical principles to the issues of euthanasia and assisted suicide.

ICEBREAKER
Death is often seen as a taboo subject. Why do you think this is?

▶ WATCH THE DVD

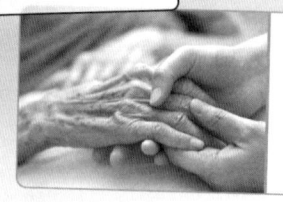

▷ END OF LIFE:
HOW SHOULD LIFE END?
Opening verses: Job 19:25–27

END OF LIFE

DVD KEY POINTS

Death is seen as 'the ultimate taboo'. Today people seem to fear the dying process more than death itself.

Approaches to death
- Fighting death
- Denial
- Despair
- Palliative treatment
- Control

Euthanasia is being killed by a doctor; assisted suicide is being helped to kill oneself. Both are currently illegal in Britain.

Life after death?
A person's greatest need is not physical health but a restored relationship with God.

Heaven and Hell put any earthly suffering into an eternal perspective.

Biblical principles
- Genesis 1–2 teaches us humans are unique, all belong to God, they must not be unjustly killed.
- 'You shall not murder'. God forbids intentional killing of the innocent.
- The Bible has no provision for 'compassionate killing'.
- The Bible does not recognise a 'right to die'.

Three mistaken positions
- 'God's law doesn't apply any more'
- 'God's law bows to God's love'
- Striving to sustain life at all costs

Palliative care acknowledges the inevitability of death, and seeks to address the needs of the dying patient.

Summary
We will not despair in the face of death because we have the hope of something far better, beyond the grave.

THE HUMAN JOURNEY

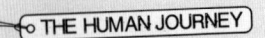

EXPLORE

Key passages: Exodus 20:13; Job 19:20, 25–27
Use these, and any other relevant passages you can think of, to help you discuss the following questions.

1 Several countries have now legalised euthanasia in one form or another. What do you think has led to this?

2 What does the Bible say about attitudes to intentional killing? Is there ever a reason to make an exception to this?

3 What hope does Christian faith offer in the face of death?

END OF LIFE

4 How should the Bible's teaching on what happens after death affect our views on euthanasia and assisted suicide?

5 If the situation arose, what would you say to a friend or relative who was considering ending their life through assisted suicide or euthanasia?

THE HUMAN JOURNEY

GO FURTHER

- Think of ways you can raise awareness about the risks and dangers of euthanasia. Perhaps you could write a letter to your MP or elected representative, post something on social media or just talk to your friends about it.

- How could you support and pray for those who are disabled, elderly or terminally ill in your church and community?

PRAY

Pray together or in smaller groups about what you've learned in this session. You may like to use these points as a guide:

- Pray for those near the end of their life and for their families.

- Pray that our lawmakers and those working in healthcare would resist the pressure to endorse or practise euthanasia.

END OF LIFE

GLOSSARY

- **Assisted suicide**: The act of helping somebody to take their own life.

- **Euthanasia**: Intentionally ending the life of someone (usually when they are very ill or in pain) with the aim of relieving their suffering. They may or may not wish to die.

- **Palliative care**: Specialised medical care for people with serious illnesses, with the aim of making the end of their life as comfortable as possible.

To continue thinking about the topics raised in this session read chapter six of *The Human Journey* book: 'End of Life – How should life end?'

More resources on End of Life are available at *www.humanjourney.org.uk*

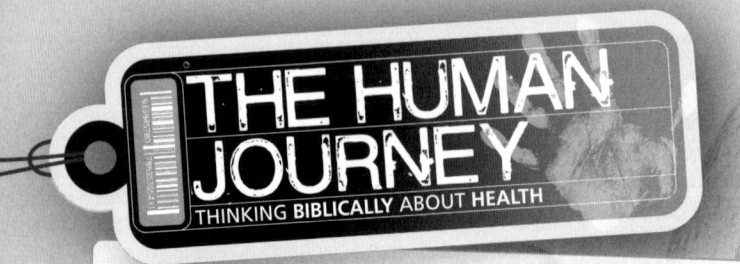

THE HUMAN JOURNEY
THINKING BIBLICALLY ABOUT HEALTH

NEW TECHNOLOGIES
ARE WE PLAYING GOD?

SESSION AIM
To understand the risks and benefits of new technological developments, and use biblical principles to consider how we should assess them.

ICEBREAKER
Imagine yourself as a 120-year-old. What would your life be like? How might the world have changed?

○─ WATCH THE DVD

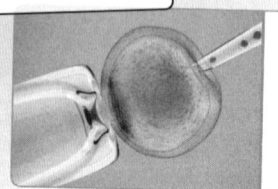

▷ NEW TECHNOLOGIES:
ARE WE PLAYING GOD?
Opening verses: Genesis 11:3–8

NEW TECHNOLOGIES

DVD KEY POINTS

New technology is dramatically impacting healthcare and lifestyles. We have embryo selection, pre-implantation genetic diagnosis, embryonic cloning, genetic engineering, animal-human hybrids, three-parent embryos.

These are often justified on the grounds that they will prevent human suffering.

'Remaking', 'faking' and 'taking' life

What does the Bible say?
- Genesis 1 – God makes human beings stewards over the whole of creation
- Genesis 4 – The development of scientific knowledge and technology

Christianity and science
- Many great scientists were Christians (eg Sir Francis Bacon, Kepler, Mendel)
- Many great doctors were Christians (eg Paré, Jenner, Simpson)

Good and bad uses of technology
- Noah builds the Ark (Genesis 6–8)
- Tower of Babel (Genesis 11)

Nine biblical principles:
- Be like the men of Issachar (1 Chronicles 12:32)
- Don't rely on the world's principles
- Hold onto truth and unity (John 17:17, 22)
- Embrace a biblical view of humanity (Genesis 1:27)
- Recognise the limits
- Keep an eternal perspective
- Embrace a wider love ('Who is my neighbour?' Luke 10:29)
- Don't let ends justify means (Romans 3:8, 6:1–2)
- Focus on the cross (Philippians 2:5–11)

Summary
Like Jesus we must be committed to fulfilling our role as God's stewards, to use our God-given gifts and abilities in God's way to help provide just and compassionate solutions for human suffering whatever it may cost.

THE HUMAN JOURNEY

EXPLORE

Key passages: Genesis 1:26–28; Genesis 11:1–9
Use these, and any other relevant passages you can think of, to help you discuss the following questions.

1 How are new medical technological developments viewed in society and reported in the press? What view of science does this promote?

2 What kind of attitude did the people have in building the Tower of Babel? What's wrong with that? Have you seen this attitude in society today?

3 What do you think we can learn about the use of technology from the story of the Tower of Babel?

NEW TECHNOLOGIES

4 How should we decide when a development in medical technology is worthwhile and when it is not?

5 'Metal may be employed to make pruning hooks and ploughshares to feed a hungry world. But it can equally be fashioned into spears and swords to kill.'

Should we ever put any technological developments 'out of bounds' or is it more a case of using all technology wisely?

6 Should Christians make use of technology that has been developed through unethical research (eg research carried out on embryos)?

THE HUMAN JOURNEY

GO FURTHER

- Talk to friends about the uses and abuses of new technologies.

- Ask someone to speak at your church on the ethical and moral challenges of a particular new technology.

- Decide on the principles you will personally employ about using new technologies in your own life.

PRAY

Pray all together or in smaller groups about what you've learned in this session. You may like to use these points as a guide:

- Give thanks that technological advances make it possible to treat previously fatal conditions.

- Ask for God to restrain human arrogance in developing technologies just because they are possible.

- Pray for Christians to be a voice of wisdom and restraint in the use of technology.

NEW TECHNOLOGIES

GLOSSARY

- **Biotechnology**: The use of living systems and organisms to develop or make products deemed to be useful.

- **In vitro fertilisation (IVF)**: a process by which an egg is fertilised by sperm outside the body (in a laboratory). Usually a number of embryos are created, and a maximum of two are implanted while the rest are frozen or destroyed.

- **Pre-implantation genetic diagnosis (PGD)**: Genetic profiling of embryos produced using IVF before they are implanted in the womb. This is used to identify embryos with hereditary conditions such as Down's syndrome, Huntington's disease or cystic fibrosis.

- **Stem cells**: Simple, unspecialised cells with the potential to become any other cell in the human body.

- **Surrogacy**: An arrangement where a woman carries and gives birth to a baby for a couple who are unable to conceive or carry a child themselves.

To continue thinking about the topics raised in this session read chapter seven of *The Human Journey* book: New Technologies – Are we playing God?

More resources on New Technologies are available at *www.humanjourney.org.uk*

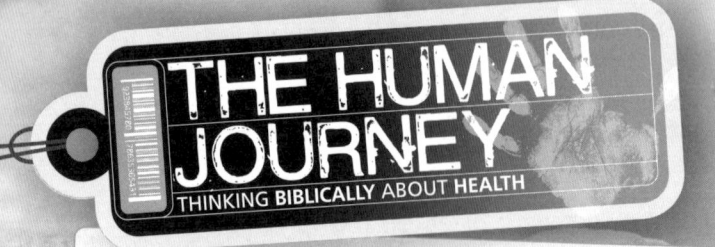

THE HUMAN JOURNEY
THINKING BIBLICALLY ABOUT HEALTH

GLOBAL HEALTH
WHO IS MY NEIGHBOUR?

SESSION AIM
To explore the differing health needs across the world and to understand Christ's call to preach the gospel and help those in need.

ICEBREAKER
What major global health issues or crises have you heard of recently? How do you feel when you hear about these and similar situations?

◦ WATCH THE DVD

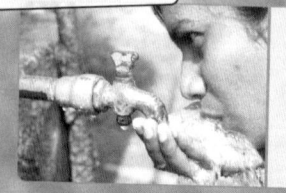

▷ GLOBAL HEALTH:
WHO IS MY NEIGHBOUR?
Opening verses: Isaiah 61:1–2

GLOBAL HEALTH

DVD KEY POINTS

In high income countries most people die of chronic diseases; in low income countries most people die of infectious diseases.

Jesus sent out his followers 'to preach the kingdom of God and to heal the sick' (Luke 9:1–2).

Jesus' describes his mission in his 'Nazareth Manifesto' (Luke 4:14–21).

Preaching
'To preach good news to the poor'
Unreached peoples are mainly in the 10:40 window – much of Africa and Asia.

Healing
'Recovery of sight for the blind'
Jesus' restoration of the whole body was a sign of the gospel's authenticity and an act of compassion.

Deliverance
'He has sent me to proclaim freedom for the prisoners'
Jesus set people free from enslaving lifestyles and circumstances.

Justice
'To release the oppressed and to proclaim the year of the Lord's favour'
Radical discipleship involves God's people bringing justice, speaking out, being advocates for and empowering vulnerable people.

The Good Samaritan (Luke 10:25-37) answers the question: 'who is my neighbour?'

Summary
Christian health professionals have huge opportunities to 'preach and heal' in the needy half of the world. But whole churches and whole Christians communities can help by praying, giving and serving in a multitude of ways.

THE HUMAN JOURNEY

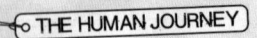

EXPLORE

Key passages: Luke 4:16–21, 10:25–37; Isaiah 58:6–12
Use these, and any other relevant passages you can think of, to help you discuss the following questions.

1 Why is the gospel 'good news for the poor?' Is God biased towards the poor? Why or why not?

2 The 'Nazareth manifesto' describes a multi-dimensional mission. Why do you think this is?

3 In what ways is the church carrying out this mission? Does anything need to change?

GLOBAL HEALTH

4 What role do you think healthcare should play in world mission today?

5 In what ways can Christians be involved in Global Health – both those who are healthcare professionals and those who are not?

6 Who is your neighbour in today's global village? How can you be a good neighbour to those in your local community and those in other countries? Can you do both?

THE HUMAN JOURNEY

GO FURTHER

- Watch or read today's news. Use this to help you pray for the world. You may find resources provided by organisations such as Operation World and Tearfund helpful in guiding your prayers.

- What has challenged you as you worked through this session? Is there something you plan to do as a result? Tell someone in the group and ask them to hold you accountable to your plan.

PRAY

Pray all together or in smaller groups about what you've learned in this session. You may like to use these points as a guide:

- Pray for a renewed desire to love your neighbour as yourself.

- Pray for Christian churches, missions and charities serving the poor at home and abroad.

- Pray for governments that they would consider those in poverty when forming new laws and policies.

GLOSSARY

- **10:40 Window**: The rectangular area between 10 and 40 degrees north of the equator (encompassing Saharan and Northern Africa, and almost all of Asia). The window is home to the majority of the world's unevangelised countries.

- **Low income countries**: Countries with a gross national income (GNI) of $1,035 or less per person (eg Afghanistan, Uganda, Cambodia, Zimbabwe).

- **High income countries**: Countries with a gross national income (GNI) of $12,616 or more per person (eg Germany, France, United States of America, United Kingdom).

To continue thinking about the topics raised in this session read chapter eight of *The Human Journey* book: Global Health – Who is my neighbour?

More resources on Global Health are available at *www.humanjourney.org.uk*

NOTES

NOTES

NOTES

NOTES